Me[n]
Midlife Challenge

Mary Batchelor

A LION BOOK

Text copyright © 1989 Mary Batchelor
This edition copyright © 1989 Lion Publishing

Published by
Lion Publishing plc
Sandy Lane West, Littlemore, Oxford, England
ISBN 0 7459 1601 5
Albatross Books Pty Ltd
PO Box 320, Sutherland, NSW 2232, Australia
ISBN 0 7324 0058 9

First edition 1989
10 9 8 7 6 5 4 3 2 1

Acknowledgments
Photographs on pages 9 and 28 by the Image Bank.
All other photographs by Zefa (UK) Ltd.

Printed and bound in Slovenia

CONTENTS

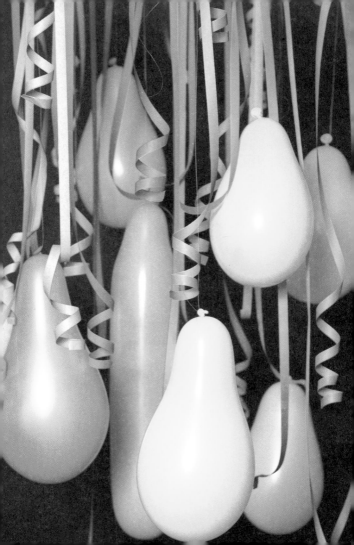

Taking Up the Challenge

'Being forty was fine,' Barry said. 'The family gave me a party and all my friends made a great fuss. It's being forty-one that's such a let-down!'

When Brigitte Bardot reached fifty, she told reporters, 'People who say it's marvellous to be fifty must be mad! It's really difficult growing old. It's not only the end of youth that gets me. It's the beginning of all the problems with health.'

Plenty of people feel the way she did. Most of us have a few qualms when we reach midlife. And it's not just health that worries us. At forty — or fifty — we come up against the whole business of leaving youth behind and facing another phase of life. We may feel anxious too about so-called midlife problems that loom ahead.

But a lot of the things about midlife that worry us beforehand may never even happen. At the very worst, no one has to cope with all the troubles that are sometimes associated with this stage in life.

On the contrary, many can say from experience

that the middle years bring a full share of enjoyment, excitement and fun. At the same time we may need courage and resources to cope with the difficulties that crop up. These may have to do with health, work, relationships in the family, or facing the future alone. They may also tie in with adjusting to getting older and leaving our youth behind.

There is a positive and a negative way to face midlife. It's fairly normal to feel some sadness and depression for a time, as we calculate the losses that seem to go with passing forty. Working through loss — of beauty, health, children or life partner — is painful.

The important thing is not to remain negative. Once we have reckoned up what we are losing, we need to look at what we stand to gain. The second half of life is different from the first half, but it can be just as good and even better. Plenty of older people will tell you that's a fact.

If we expect midlife to be a total disaster, the prophecy is likely to be fulfilled. It's far better to treat midlife as a challenge. It's a time of life we can welcome and enjoy. It's a time to develop new strengths, new growth as a person, and a new zest for living.

Bridging the Gap

'I feel as though I'm always the one in the middle,' one 47-year-old woman said. She had to cope with teenage daughters and two younger children, as well as caring for her elderly mother and mother-in-law, who both lived nearby.

Many people in midlife find themselves looking after two generations — their children and their parents too.

Midlife may bring greater demands at work. Most people of forty and over are under pressure from those higher up the career ladder, as well as from younger men and women climbing up behind.

People in midlife are likely to have heavy responsibilities. They often have key jobs in the community. In the middle years we can really feel *caught* in the middle.

There's another and better way of looking at the situation.

'I see the people in midlife as the bridge generation,' a forty-year-old man said. 'It's a terrific privilege to be the ones who influence and lead.'

It helps when we take this positive viewpoint. It means we don't see ourselves as helpless victims. We are the people in control. We are at the heart of our families and our communities, able to use our experience and skills to support and guide the generations on either side.

Because of the responsibility we carry, we are likely to get tired and to find life demanding.

'However long I try to stay with Dad, he always complains when I go,' one woman sighed. 'I really should be at home getting dinner for the family. The trouble is, I just don't know how to divide my time or decide who needs me most.'

Sometimes, within the family, the job seems to bring very little reward.

'Whatever I say is wrong,' one mother of a teenage son lamented.

Another woman admitted sadly, 'My mother always grumbles. I never seem to do quite what she had hoped I would.'

But life is also hard for the teenagers and the elderly people we are trying to help. It's natural that they should sometimes be cross and touchy. Even when they grumble and complain, they still need us to love them. They want us to show our love, not just by doing the chores, but by accepting them as they are and understanding their needs.

Real love is tough and costly. A famous chapter in the New Testament describes love as 'slow to lose patience. It looks for a way of being constructive.

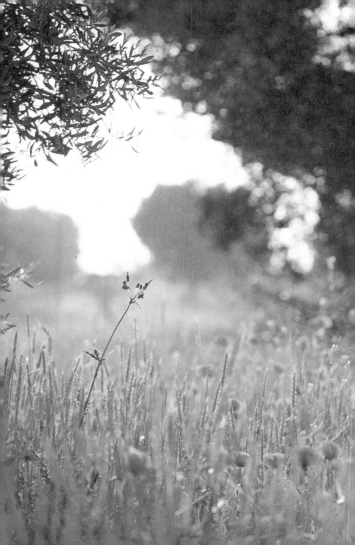

Dealing with the Past

'I can remember the day . . . '

'When we were children we used to . . . '

By the time we reach midlife, we have stored up many memories, happy and sad. Some begin with the words, 'I wish I hadn't.' They are usually ones we would rather forget. In fact we sometimes bury these memories deep within us because we can't bring ourselves to remember things that make us ashamed and disgusted with ourselves.

When we do something wrong we harm someone — either other people or ourselves. Wrongdoing goes deep. It damages us as individuals. We don't escape the long-term effects.

The Bible tells us of a time when David, Israel's greatest king, committed adultery and murder. When he realized the enormity of what he had done, he made a rather surprising statement. His sin, he said, was not primarily against the woman he had seduced or the man he had had killed. It was against God. David knew that wrongdoing not only damages our relationship with others, it also injures our relationship with God.

God made us for himself. It is his plan that we should find purpose and happiness in life through loving and obeying him. But every time we choose to go our own way and please ourselves we sin against him and need his forgiveness. We have driven a wedge between ourselves and God.

But God does not simply write us off. He wants to give us the chance to put things right and begin again. The good news is that he sent his son, Jesus Christ, into our world to make forgiveness and new life possible.

Once God has forgiven us, we may need to ask forgiveness from other people we have hurt. Midlife is a good time to set the past to rights and make a fresh start with the new quality of life that God can give us.

A middle-aged woman was telling a friend how badly someone had treated her. She ended bitterly, 'Whatever happens, I'll never forgive her!' Jesus told his followers that those who want God to forgive them must be ready to forgive others. Asking forgiveness is one side of a coin, offering forgiveness is the other. The two must go together.

Holding on to hatred and resentment makes us bitter and hard. When we know the happiness and freedom that God's forgiveness brings, we have the best possible reason for forgiving those who have wronged us.

'I want to forgive my husband, but I can't,'

one woman told me after her divorce. But she
was half-way there. When we can honestly tell
God that we are willing *to forgive, he is ready to*
help us do it.

Whatever mess we may have made of life so far,
God is prepared to start all over again with us. He
can heal the hurts of the past. He can begin now,
in this life, to create something — *someone* — new
and worthwhile.

Planning for the Future

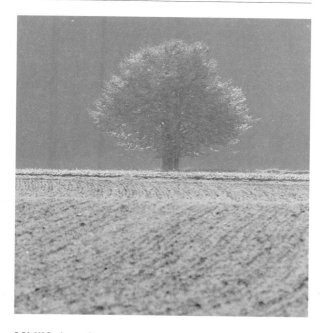

Midlife is a time when we begin to think about the future in a new way. We realize that youth is past; middle age and old age lie ahead. As we picture the problems the new stages in life may bring, we are often afraid. Our fears take many different forms.

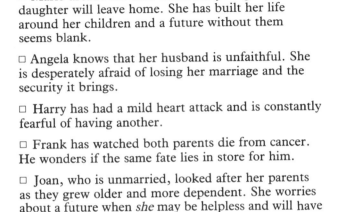

☐ Donald has arthritis. He wonders how long he will be able to cope with the rush-hour travel to work and the physical demands of his job.

☐ Marie dreads the time when her youngest daughter will leave home. She has built her life around her children and a future without them seems blank.

☐ Angela knows that her husband is unfaithful. She is desperately afraid of losing her marriage and the security it brings.

☐ Harry has had a mild heart attack and is constantly fearful of having another.

☐ Frank has watched both parents die from cancer. He wonders if the same fate lies in store for him.

☐ Joan, who is unmarried, looked after her parents as they grew older and more dependent. She worries about a future when *she* may be helpless and will have have no one to care for her.

Not one of these people is likely to talk about his or her fears. It can often help to know that others share our worries, but we don't readily discuss them because we feel that it is weak or immature to be frightened.

An active imagination can be a mixed blessing. Many of the events we picture in our minds never happen. But even when they do, they bring with them compensations and strengths that we cannot know about in advance.

We usually find that the ordeals of the next day, dreaded as we lie awake the night before, are easier to cope with once the time arrives. The sleepless hours of worry actually make us less fit to cope. Jesus reminded his followers that worry never makes the slightest difference to a problem. He advised them to leave tomorrow to look after itself. Today's problems are quite enough for today.

There is an even better reason for not worrying about the future. God is a strong and loving Father, who knows all about our needs. He knows every detail of what lies ahead for us and for those we love. We can tell him about our most intimate fears and leave the working out of our future in his capable hands.

God has promised to care for his children whatever their age. He says, 'I am your God and will take care of you until you are old and your hair is grey. I made you and I will care for you; I will give you help and rescue you.'

We don't have to wait until we are old to take comfort from that promise. It can help us here and now to put our fears about the future into true perspective.

Gateway to Life

When we reach midlife we may experience the loss of parents, aunts and uncles, or even husband or wife. Death comes close to us, perhaps for the first time.

Bereavement brings mixed emotions. We may experience guilt and anger as well as numbness. The pain and the sense of loss may last for a very long while.

It is hard at first to realize the finality of what has taken place. It can take a long time to come to terms with the fact that we shall never again see the person whose life was so bound up with our own.

There are many ways of trying to deal with grief and loss. I recently read a book written to help children cope with the death of someone close. The writer reminded them that the person they loved would live on in the memory of their friends.

However, there is a deeper source of comfort than that. It is possible for hope and joy to be stronger even than grief. God has shown us through Jesus' resurrection that death is not the end. Jesus promised his followers, 'Because I live, you too will live.' A person who dies trusting in Jesus does not cease to exist, but enjoys full life and joy with God, free from pain and sadness.

The death of someone close can shake us. The whole stable framework of life now looks frail and temporary. Nothing and no one seems safe any more.

In the seventeenth century, John Donne wrote: 'Ask not for whom the bell tolls. It tolls for thee.' The passing of someone close reminds us forcibly of our own mortality. When we are young, we think we are immortal. By midlife, an event that had seemed remote and unreal becomes an inescapable fact. We calculate that we have already used up half our allotted life span.

One writer states that all of us must come to terms with the fact of our own death, and then get on with living life. But she gives no clues about how to do so!

Some people opt out. They continue to put the thought out of their minds, hoping that if they ignore death it will go away. It won't. We prepare carefully for every other important event of life. How much more should we prepare for our own death. That does not mean dwelling on it morbidly. It means thinking again about our beliefs and considering what we need to do *now* in order to be ready for death when it comes.

Jesus offers us a new kind of life. It begins here, in the present, and continues and expands beyond death. It is called eternal life, because it is the kind of life that God, the Eternal One, possesses.

Jesus promises eternal life to all who give their lives into his keeping. Using picture language, he said, 'I give my sheep eternal life, and they shall never die.' Under the guiding, caring leadership of the good shepherd, death is not the end of the road. It is the gateway to life.

New Goals

When I was fifty I went through a difficult time. We moved to a new house just as the children were leaving home for good, and that made me feel as if my whole life as I'd known it for the past twenty-five years had come to an end. The future looked like a downhill path, leading nowhere and without purpose.

Negative feelings about the future are common at midlife. Many of the aims we started out with at twenty or thirty no longer fit. Those early ambitions had to do with choosing a career, making money, finding a life partner, raising a family, having a home and making a place for ourselves in the world. By the time we are forty-five or fifty we have either achieved these aims or abandoned them as no longer appropriate.

Some people feel a sense of failure because their ambitions have come to nothing. Relationships have gone sour. The longed-for children never arrived. Or their children have not turned out as the parents hoped. Disappointments may have come at work:

little recognition; no advancement; inadequate
reward.

Others have achieved many of the things they
set out to do. Their marriages have survived, their
children are successfully launched, they have
reached the position they hoped for at work, and
they have made enough money to live comfortably.

Both kinds of people can feel lost and empty
at midlife.

Human beings need something to aim at and strive
for. When we reach the end of the programme we
mapped out for ourselves years before, we are left
without purpose. All the important milestones seem
to be behind us. It's not surprising that many people
begin to ask:

'Is this all there is?'

'Is there any point in going on?'

'What is left to look forward to?'

The fact that early goals have been achieved, or
else abandoned as impossible, in no way means that
the game is over. The second half of life calls for new
goals suited to the new stage we have reached.

For those who missed the chance to prepare for a
chosen career, now may be the time to begin. With
the family off their hands, men may be able to afford
to take time off for training and women may be
freer to do so.

Others may prefer to find alternative outlets for
their interests and abilities. A would-be teacher

can help with voluntary care of small children; a frustrated nurse can train in first-aid duties.

Sometimes we need to turn in a new direction. Some men and women achieve this about-turn by launching into a new career in midlife. They see the need to develop a side of themselves that has been smothered in the earlier years. For example, a clerical worker might use untapped creative skills by becoming a cook or artist. A computer specialist might change to a job that involves caring for people.

Even without changing jobs, many people are able to correct the balance of their lives. They may resolve to think less of making money and more of fostering relationships within the family and community. Women who have been kept busy at home may be able to widen the scope of their care, using the experience they have gained over the years. Those who have ignored or suppressed the spiritual side of their nature may resolve to correct that vital balance. They may explore the spiritual dimension through reading and through prayer. They may discover the Bible for themselves.

Life really can begin at forty or fifty, or even later. There is so much to enjoy and to give to others, provided we realign our aims and set new goals.

Celebrating Midlife

'I never expected I'd enjoy getting older,' Katy
admitted. 'The best thing is that I feel free!'
Katy's children have left home and her husband,
who took early retirement, is doing part-time work.
'It seems such a luxury to be able to plan my day
without fixing everything around Jack's job and the
family's programme. I never thought middle age
would be so good!'

Linda has cashed in on her new situation in the
same way. For many years she combined a job with
looking after her elderly mother. She used to come
home from the office in the lunch hour every day,
and even took her mother on holiday with her. Then
her mother died. Linda realized that she was free
now to do all the things she had previously been able
only to watch from the side lines. She still spends
some of her free time visiting and caring for elderly
people — she understands their needs — but she has
also begun taking evening classes and is learning to
ski. She is freer now than when she was thirty.

Midlife can set us free in other ways. When we

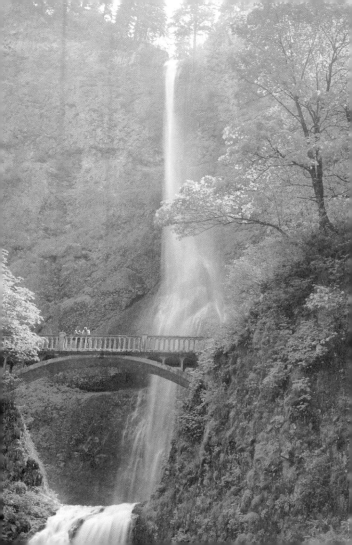

It is not possessive. It knows no limit to its endurance . . . it can outlast anything.' That is the kind of love that God offers *us*. For many it is a lifeline.

Sometimes we lose patience with the people we are helping. We may feel like giving up hope. But when we reach out in love — the kind of love that tries to understand, accept, and find a way through — we may make a success of being the generation in the middle.

3

'It's My Age!'

'I can remember what my mother was like during the menopause. I only hope I don't go through what she did!'

Quite a few women have memories like that. When they get to their forties they begin to wonder what is in store for them, and how they will cope.

There's probably no need for them to worry. Of course the hormone changes that mark the end of the childbearing years *may* affect the emotions as well as the body. But nowadays those who find it difficult to carry on normally can get medical treatment that really helps.

A good number of women sail through with few, if any, problems. One woman said: 'I asked my doctor if there's something wrong with me, because I've got through the menopause without any trouble!'

Most are affected only mildly. And all can take comfort from the fact that the problems are relatively short-term.

Once the menopause is over, many women feel fitter and better able to cope, at work and in their family life, than they have ever done before.

It's not only women who worry about their health in midlife. Men also have various anxieties and minor ailments.

Some people worry about disease. Is my blood pressure or heart normal? Could I have cancer? It's important to deal with fears like these, even if they turn out to be groundless. So if you *are* worried, arrange for a medical check-up.

It is of course wise to take practical steps to keep fit. Give up smoking, cut down on alcohol, and change to a healthy diet. Get regular exercise. That will make you feel better, and there will be less need to worry about your health!

It's important, however, to adapt to the new stage of life and stop working and playing as if you were still twenty.

For a small minority, this time of life means facing up to pain and disability that will not go away. If this is your situation, it is important to go on doing the things you enjoy. But you will need to pace yourself, to allow proper time for rest, and to think how ordinary tasks can be made easier in practical ways.

Midlife is often a time of unsettled feelings. Our moods change quickly, and we may get depressed. That's perfectly normal. It will pass, once we have adjusted to this new stage in life.

In the meantime, people close to us may wonder why we are irritable or seem somehow different from usual. More than one husband has said to his wife, 'You're not the woman I married.' Wives may wonder what has changed their husbands too. It's hard to cope with misunderstanding from those close to us when we're having trouble understanding ourselves.

What helped me was realizing that God knows me through and through, whether or not I understood myself. A psalm in the Bible says: 'Lord, you know me. You know everything I do; from far away you understand all my thoughts. You see me, whether I am working or resting — you are all around me on every side; you protect me with your power — you created every part of me.'

God not only understands us, he cares about us too.

4

Pressure Points

'I feel as if something inside my head is going to burst!'

'If he says another word, I'll scream!'

'I've had it up to here!'

You don't have to be going through a midlife crisis to feel like that, but the middle years often coincide with the extra stress and tensions that lead to such outbursts.

Hormone changes may affect moods and emotions. Heavy periods or bad nights may leave us feeling constantly tired. Having to cope with a load of extra responsibility at work and with the family can make us edgy and tense.

It's not just hard work that tires us. There are many difficult decisions to make at this stage of life. Some of them concern us and some have to do with the people who depend on us in our jobs or at home.

Strain and anxiety make us tense and can affect

our health. So can trying to pack in more than will possibly fit into twenty-four hours. Somehow we need to find a way to manage the situation. Lying awake at night worrying is certainly not the answer.

The first step is to look for ways to cut down the actual workload. For example, other members of the family could take a turn at caring for an elderly relative, or share in difficult decisions about the future.

Talking things over with someone who is close to us, or who has been trained to help, may ease the burden too.

It is important to use our time and energy in the best possible way. Make a list of all your regular jobs — then cross off any that aren't absolutely necessary. Decide on the basis that people matter more than things.

No matter how many cuts we make, we shall still have limited time to give to the people who need us. But quality counts more than quantity in human relationships. However short the time we have to spend, what matters to the person we are with is giving them our full attention while we are there. That's especially important to an elderly parent, or a teenage son or daughter.

When I give all my attention to the person I am with, instead of letting my mind wander on to all the jobs that have still to be done, it not only helps the other person — it also frees *me* from stress and tension.

When life is demanding and busy, it is natural to

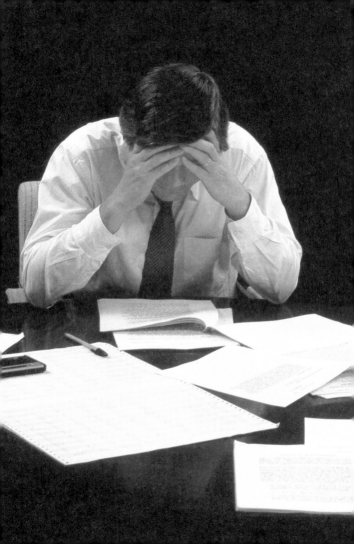

try to spend every waking moment coping with the extra workload. A better solution is to take time out to relax. Exercise — even just walking — restores the mind as well as the body. To relax flat out on the floor, even for ten minutes, can work wonders.

It's hard to stop doing things and be still when there are so many jobs to be done. But I try to follow this good advice: 'Build into your day little enclosures of silence; they spill over into your life and bring peace, the peace of God.'

5

Someone Who Matters

'My parents are dead, and I don't feel as if I matter to anyone now.'

'My husband's left me for someone half my age. Who cares now if I'm alive or dead?'

'The children have their own lives to live. They don't need me any more.'

People don't always put thoughts like those into words, but that's the way they sometimes feel when they get to midlife. If there is no one they are especially close to, or who seems to need them, they feel as if they no longer count.

Others get hard knocks at work. They think they don't matter because they haven't made a success of their job. 'I put everything I had into my work and then the other man was promoted.' Or perhaps they give years of loyal service only to be given the push when the work force is cut. No wonder their self-esteem is at rock bottom!

Part of the trouble is that we take our values from those around us. Our society seems to say that to count for anything we must be successful, and success is reckoned in terms of money, possessions, status and what looks — at least from the outside — like a good share of fun and happiness.

It might surprise us to discover that the most successful people we know are having similar self-doubts at this time of life. Men and women who have money, or who have reached the top of their career, often feel cheated too. The prizes they worked so hard for don't satisfy.

The happy families we look at wistfully probably have their own share of difficulties and failure too. We don't tell others all *our* private troubles, and so we don't realize how common these feelings of failure can be.

Midlife is often a time of loss. A partner may leave, or children go away from home. A parent may die. Loss is always painful. It often reduces our confidence too. We don't feel we matter any more.

We can't hurry the process of regaining our self-esteem. But it helps to know that midlife is a time of change for everyone. Given time, we *will* emerge again with confidence, worthwhile commitments and a new sense of purpose.

This renewed confidence doesn't always come about automatically, however. We have to begin looking for ways to fill the empty spaces, gradually building up a new life and a new sense of worth.

Each of us does *matter. A lot of people need us. Our world is crying out for people who care and are prepared to shoulder some of the hard work*

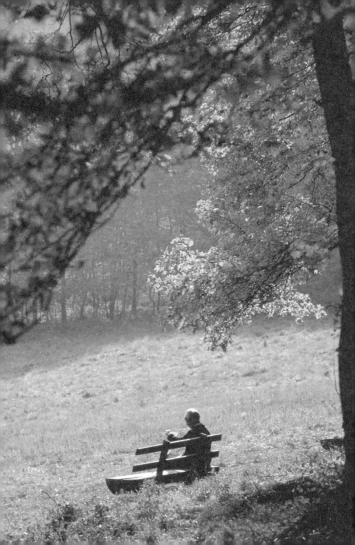

of meeting others' needs. There is plenty of scope in every community.

When we reach out to others and offer them help and love, we do more to help ourselves than when we concentrate on our own needs and try to make ourselves happy.

There is a deeper reason for believing that we matter. God, who made us, is totally concerned and involved with us. He is not some kind of far-off First Principle, letting the world run on in its own way. He is a loving Father, who knows all our needs and who wants the best for us. God does not demand that we bring him a list of achievements. He loves us *as we are.*

6

Who Am I?

'They used to call me that woman with all the children,' Jenny said. 'I didn't mind — I loved being a mother. Now all four of them have left home, and we've moved. Lots of people here don't even know I have children. And I don't seem to know who I am any more.'

Jack ran the local store until he had to retire early because of illness. He has something in common with Jenny. 'I used to know who I was. I was known in the town. Now I feel I've lost my identity.'

Most of us are used to being known by our labels. We're someone's daughter or aunt or boss. We're the teacher's wife, the butcher or the librarian. We usually take it for granted that people need to label us in order to file us away in their memories.

Sometimes the label becomes our reason for living. Instead of seeing it as a job description we use it to define ourselves as people. Some women label themselves *wife* or *mother* for most of their adult lives. Some men and women are so immersed in their jobs that they begin to think they *are* what they *do*.

The trouble begins when the label has to be dropped and they are left with no other identity. When a husband walks out, children leave home, a parent dies or the job finishes, a crisis follows. Sometimes there doesn't seem to be a real person behind the label. Men and women, shocked and stripped of their reason for living, begin to ask, 'Who am I?' 'What is the point of life?'

The truth is that we are bigger than any of the jobs we do. Behind every label stands a real person. Having the label removed can be the first step towards discovering who we really are.

One woman who had been divorced described one positive gain from her painful experience: 'I married very young and felt that I must always say and do what my husband wanted. I wasn't being myself, but trying to be the person he expected. Now I'm learning to be myself for the first time.'

Finding our real identity means coming to terms with our strengths and weaknesses. It means being true to ourselves, rather than using our label in order to impress people. We may be forced to find the courage to stand alone. We may have to let go of the emotional ties that bind us to our family.

Each of us needs to recognize that we matter because we are unique individuals, created by God. We don't have to borrow status from job, possessions, friends or family.

It is true that a sense of identity is linked with belonging — to a nation, a community, a family. Cutting off our roots and trying to do without any

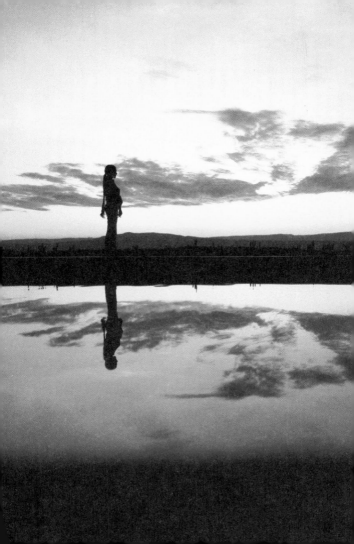

identifying label is not the way to find our true selves. We need to belong — *and yet be free to be ourselves.*

God describes his people as a family and himself as Father. He invites each one of us into his family, where we can experience a special sense of belonging. But it is not a new kind of identity trap. When we turn to God and refocus our lives, we become truly free to be ourselves.

7

Marriage Matters

Is it reasonable to expect a marriage to last a lifetime, now that it may mean spending fifty or sixty years together? Many people think not. But marriage can in fact be a loving, growing partnership that continues to nourish and help both partners as the years go by.

Whatever our views, a good many marriages *do* break down sooner or later, and statistics show certain high-risk periods. Midlife is one of them.

Perhaps that isn't surprising. Midlife is often a time of self-doubt and emotional upheaval. This easily spills over into the marriage. Just when they need each other most, husband and wife may find it almost impossible to share their deepest thoughts and feelings or to express their fears and needs.

There are other reasons why marriages break down in midlife. Some couples stick together until the family is off their hands or until parents, who would be badly hurt, are dead. Then they feel free to make the break.

Marriages can also founder at this stage because the

partners are too busy. Couples may be stretched to the limit with demanding jobs as well as family cares. They don't make time to foster and strengthen their relationship.

Boredom as well as neglect can kill a marriage. When the children leave home, some couples have nothing to say to each other. On the physical side, they may have made no effort to explore and discover sex that satisfies them both. Routine and lack of effort make any relationship boring. So do selfishness and a failure to think of the other partner's needs.

After ten or twenty years or more, there is a danger that husband and wife will take each other for granted. Neither troubles to say 'thank you' or to appreciate what the other one does.

Without even realizing what she is doing, a wife may steadily undermine her husband's confidence by nagging and negative comments.

The husband may be painfully aware that he is not so young or successful as he would like to be. He may also be afraid that he is losing his sexual powers. When a younger woman who clearly admires him comes along, it can be balm to the husband's ego.

In the same way, a woman who has been taken for granted at home may blossom and feel that she is a person in her own right when she is listened to and complimented by another man.

It's easy to see how an affair can be sparked off, or even why a husband or wife may want a permanent change of partner. But is that the answer to dissatisfactions within the marriage?

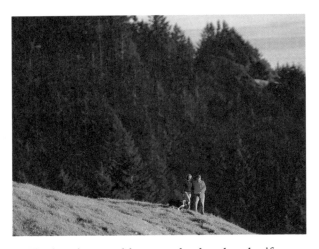

The bond created between husband and wife
is too strong to be put aside without great pain
and personal damage. Unfaithfulness and marriage
breakdown bring deep sadness and loss to almost all
the people involved. Not only the marriage partners
but children, grandparents and parents suffer too.

God designed marriage to be a lifelong faithful
relationship between husband and wife. That is the
ideal. If a marriage is to last, there must be total
commitment and a real concern for the partner's
happiness and the good of the whole family. Couples
need to be unselfish and persevering if the early
romantic joy-ride is to become a satisfying journey
together through life.

Midlife is an ideal time for a couple to take a new

look at their relationship. When both are honest and want to please and help each other, the relationship can change, adjusting to every new phase of life.

Marriage is God's invention — and he will help couples keep their marriage healthy and alive, even through the difficult years of midlife.

8

All by Myself

Many people, women more than men, face midlife on their own. Some who have stayed single and live at home or nearby may lose their parents. Others are widowed or coping alone after a broken marriage. As children grow up and leave home, single parents are left alone for the first time.

These days most of us live away from the bigger family circle and the friends we grew up with. So there are plenty of people who find themselves alone when they reach midlife.

It takes time to come to terms with loss through bereavement or divorce. There is no given length of time for mourning — it takes some people longer than others. Those who lose a partner in midlife are especially vulnerable. Often they have weathered the demanding years of bringing up a family and coping with money strains, and they feel bitterly cheated out of the easier years together they had looked forward to.

Single people experience problems at midlife too. Those who have never married and who thought that they had accepted their singleness may need to work through negative emotions again at this new stage. They may be plagued by doubts as to whether they could in fact have sustained a permanent relationship. Those who have had a number of sexual partners may suffer similar doubts and fears. They too may fear that years of loneliness lie ahead.

The society which we live in thinks in terms of couples, so we sometimes take it for granted that being alone is a bad thing. But there are advantages too. Those of us who never get a moment's peace at work or at home often long for a few hours on our own. Ideally, we would all like a bit of both — other people's company as well as time alone when we want it. But life doesn't usually work like that and we have to make the best of the situation we are in.

Many people living on their own enjoy the advantages. They relish the freedom to make choices without needing to refer to others who depend on them or want to have a say in decision-making. They choose friends, leisure pursuits and a daily routine to suit themselves.

Olive really enjoys planning her own timetable, but she recognizes that she can easily become insensitive to other people's needs.

Eileen, who was widowed early, says she was helped eighteen months later when a nephew came to live with her for a few months. At first she was horrified at the untidy rooms, empty fridge and dirty washing. Then she realized that he had arrived just in time to stop her getting into a narrow and selfish routine.

Those who are on their own must guard against keeping themselves to themselves, against being afraid to show love or affection in case they get hurt. For the key that unlocks the prison of loneliness is care and kindness to others.

We must look for those who need our affection and friendship if we are not to become small and shrivelled people. As we love others, our own emptiness and need for love will be met and satisfied.

It is in giving that we receive.

*are younger we have to satisfy others by behaving as
they expect and need us to. We try hard to be model
parents — or children — and to fit our work role of
secretary, salesman, or policeman. To some extent,
our personality is squeezed into the mould prepared
for us. We feel the need to conform. By midlife, we
can relax and be ourselves.*

'I don't mind any more what people think,'
Dorothy said. 'If I feel like it I sing in the
supermarket as well as in the bath. And when I
have to talk to absolute strangers, I no longer worry
about what they'll think of me. I suppose I've grown
more confident.'

Ellen, who is older, added: 'I think it's easier to
talk to men now. No one is going to think you're
flirting. You can just enjoy a good talk and a laugh
without being self-conscious. There's lots to be said
for getting older!'

*By the time we reach midlife we have gained
at least some wisdom and experience. We have had
time to develop our interests and tastes so that we
know how to select what is good. Better still, we
have learned to tell the difference between what
matters and what is not worth bothering about.*

We have discovered a good bit about our fellow
human beings too. We know whom to trust and
where to put our confidence. We value the worth
of real *friends*.

Mary has made an even more important
discovery. 'I've learned that whatever life brings,
God is with me in it. I began to trust him when I was

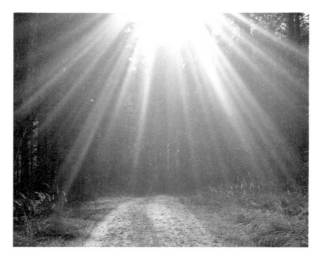

very young, but only in midlife have I really learned how much he loves me and how special I am to him. Now I'm free to love him in return, and I try to put him at the centre of my life.

'Midlife — for me — is a time to celebrate.'